BREAST AUGMENTATION
With No Scar On The Breast

WILLIAM R. BURDEN
M.D., F.A.C.S.

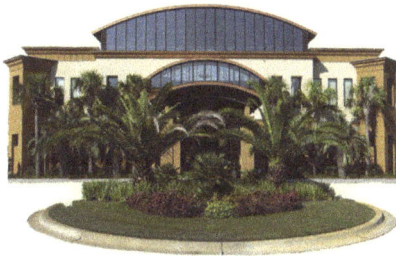

DESTIN
PLASTIC SURGERY
www.ThePlasticDoc.com

Table Of Contents

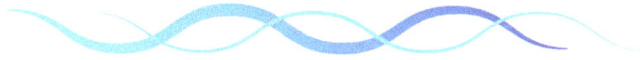

Introduction

This book is intended to be an overview of breast augmentation for women considering this procedure. Before having a consultation with a plastic surgeon, many women don't realize all of the various options and decisions which will need to be made in order to achieve their ideal breast shape and size. You will find information about various breast augmentation options in this book, focusing extensively on the No Scar on the Breast technique. I believe this technique has the highest rate of satisfaction for patients when performed by a qualified plastic surgeon.

Early Fiber Optics Research

During my fellowship in Plastic Surgery at the University of Florida in the 1990s, I was one of the first surgeons at the University of Florida researching a new approach to breast augmentation surgery using fiber optics, which allowed for a smaller incision and an incision in the underarm area. The result—no scar on the breast! During the course of this research we found that these new techniques led to a higher level of patient satisfaction with their results. My experiences in the research over twenty years ago led me to continually refine this approach and to date I have performed thousands of No Scar on the Breast procedures. In the balance of this introduction I will cover a little history because the feedback from patients in the early stages of my research formed my impressions of what patients really want when they are seeking this procedure.

During my general surgery residency, which was in the late '80s to early '90s, there was a revolution in surgery utilizing fiber optic technology. Surgeons had been performing major general surgery procedures and thoracic procedures with a large incision that allowed access to the body cavity or area for the surgery. When fiber optic technology was developed, surgeons started realizing that we could use this new technology and make smaller incisions. We could still do the procedure and the patient would have less pain during recovery. As general surgeons, we all learned how to do gallbladder surgery, lung resection surgery, appendectomies and other procedures using this revolutionary fiber optic technology.

Breast Augmentation Using Fiber Optic Technology

Many of us went on to fellowships in plastic surgery, cardiothoracic surgery and other specialties. Plastic surgeons were contemplating how to use the new fiber optic technology in their work and one area of focus was in breast augmentation. Several centers around the country started using this technology, one of which was the University of Florida.

Visible Scars Vs. Hidden Scars

During this same time there was a controversy regarding silicone implants. Due to some negative publicity, patients became frightened of silicone implants. The University of Florida was one of the large toxicology centers that focused on studies looking at the toxicology of silicone implants. Patients would come in and we would have a very extensive physical exam and questionnaire where we would ask different questions about their breast augmentation results. Part of the studies involved patients' thoughts on the results of their breast augmentation. After hearing their answer, we would also give our thoughts on the breast augmentation result.

I would see a patient who would have a very good result from her breast augmentation, and I'd ask, "What do you think of your results?" The patient might have a scar around the areola or under the breast, and maybe the scar was good, but it was visible. The patient would say, "Well, what do you think? This is a terrible result. Look at this scar." I would say, "Ma'am, your actual result is pretty good, but yes, I can see that your scar is not that favorable." The next patient would have a good result, and her incision would be under the arm. I'd ask, "Well, can I see your incision?" It might not be a very good scar. I'm thinking she's going to be complaining about her result, and she would say, "Well, my result is excellent." I'd say, "Well, what about your scar?" She'd say, "Well, no one ever sees that scar, so this is fine with me." This played out over and over again.

No Scar on the Breast Procedure Leads To Higher Satisfaction Rate

It became apparent to me that if a surgeon could achieve a consistently good result and put the incision remotely, not on the breast, the patient would be very satisfied. That prompted me to pursue the transaxillary approach more and more. With the incision in the underarm, no one complained of the appearance of a scar on the breast.

Years ago, before fiber optic technology, the underarm approach had a problem with consistent placement. Placement of the implant was performed "blindly." With fiber optic technology, we were able to put a camera into the pocket, which provided 10X magnification for superior visualization of the pocket. Under endoscopic guidance, the implant is placed more accurately than using the traditional inframammary fold approach or periareolar approach. It became very apparent that we were able to get as good or better placement, and put the scar in a remote position (in the underarm instead of on the breast).

During my fellowship we were able to refine the transaxillary incision approach. When I entered private practice in the Destin, Florida area, I offered this procedure along with the more traditional approaches. When you're in private practice, the patients, many times, request the type of incision. I would honor their request and performed breast augmentations through the different incision locations.

As time progressed, I found exactly the same thing that I had encountered in my fellowship. If a patient had a scar on her breast that did not heal as well as she thought it should, even though her breast shape was fine, she wasn't very happy. Whereas, using the transaxillary approach I have had few comments about the scar not looking good, because it is rarely seen due to the location. Over time, I've steered my patients towards this technique. I achieve a good result, highly predictable, accurate, with no scar on the breast.

QUESTIONS & ANSWERS (Q & A's)

Q: What are the most typical reasons that women consider having breast augmentation?

A: Every woman is unique and beautiful in her own way, so reasons for breast augmentation are varied. In general, this procedure is performed to increase breast volume and improve breast shape. There are many considerations, but for the majority of the patients I see, it's really for fit of the clothes. They want to look good in their bathing suit, the regular clothes they're wearing as a professional, or even as a stay-at-home mom. Rarely do I see a woman who wants to have incredibly large breasts or wants to show off her busty physique. There are a few, and that's fine if that's what they want.

In their minds, women know how they want to look. They want to match their body with their bust. A woman will look in the mirror and she knows what she wants her shape to be, and she knows how she wants her clothes to fit. If she doesn't achieve that, then she may try to do something to fill that spot. Whether it's wearing a padded bra, squeezing into a girdle, or wearing hair extensions, they will find a way. In the case where those tactics don't quite work or when they're tired of using all those camouflage techniques, then they resort to the surgery to give them that shape that they want.

Additionally, when women have had children, they lose some of their breast volume, especially if they've maintained their weight from pre-pregnancy, or have actually leaned down. They may want to get their pre-pregnancy physique back. This can be achieved with breast enhancement. Many women want to have the bust they had when nursing. Pregnancy breasts are sometimes a teaser to breast augmentation.

Breast augmentation might be right for you if you want to:

- Increase the size of naturally small breasts
- Return breasts to the size they were before weight loss
- Return breasts to the size they were before pregnancy or breastfeeding
- Balance breasts that are a different size
- Attain a full, curvy bustline
- Balance the proportion between the upper body and the hips

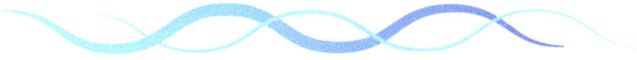

Q: ***Who are good candidates for breast enhancement?***

A: A good candidate is a woman who's in overall good health, is in reasonably good shape and has reasonable expectations for her results. She doesn't have to be in perfect health. She may have a bit of breast droop, especially after having children or weight loss and her skin may be stretched out a little bit so she's not going to have the breasts of an 18 or 19 year old, but still has a reasonable shape.

A good candidate will also understand that this is a process and the day after surgery, she will not look perfect. There will be some swelling and bruising. There will be some distortion of the shape for the first week or so. By the third or fourth week, she'll start to appreciate the improvement in her breasts. As time progresses, she'll see the results. It's really matching up the expectations with what's possible. That is a key to a woman being a good candidate for the procedure.

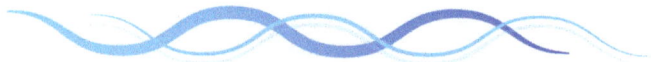

Q: *There are many options for breast augmentation. When a patient is interested in an augmentation procedure, what decisions need to be made and how do you help guide the patient in making the decisions during a consultation?*

A: Every woman is unique and your individual shape and goals will help the surgeon make suggestions for a procedure that will achieve the goals you have for your resulting breast shape after the procedure. One of the fundamental decisions is the location of the incision and thus, the location of the resulting scar. We also have a choice in types of implants, saline or silicone, as well as the shape and size, or the volume of the implants. Another important decision is the location of the implants, above or below the pectoral muscles.

One of the most critical decisions a patient can make is the choice of plastic surgeon for the procedure. Not all plastic surgeons are experienced with all of the surgical options, so you will want to make sure the surgeon you select has appropriate experience with the type procedure that you have an interest in. As an example, if you are interested in a procedure where an incision is made in the underarm, with the result being that there is no visible scar on the breast, you will want to select a surgeon with the extensive experience and access to the medical instrumentation required for such a procedure. Being one of the pioneers in this advanced technique, I have many years of experience and have performed thousands of successful procedures with this technique.

Many plastic surgeons are **not** technically capable of performing the transaxillary technique or have little experience with it. They will try to discourage you from this technique by giving you false ideas and information about the transaxillary "No Scar on the Breast" technique.

Your breast augmentation consultation is one of the most important steps you will make toward attaining the attractive shape that you desire. When you come in for your consultation, your surgeon will explain all of your available options and how the procedure is performed. Our office has state-of-the-art 3-D imaging systems so we can show you a simulation of what you might look like after surgery. This system enables you to compare implants of different sizes and types and to see the potential new you in 3-D, before surgery.

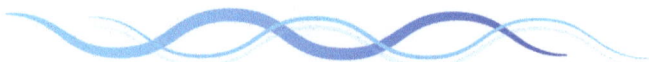

Q: Since the location of the incision determines where there will be a scar, this is an important decision. What are the various options for incision location?

A: There are three typical incision locations. These can be seen in the illustration on the next page. While the vast majority of my patients choose the transaxillary or No Scar on the Breast underarm incision, some choose incisions through the inframammary fold (IMF), which is placed in the crease beneath the breast and the periareolar incision, which runs along the lower border of the areola.

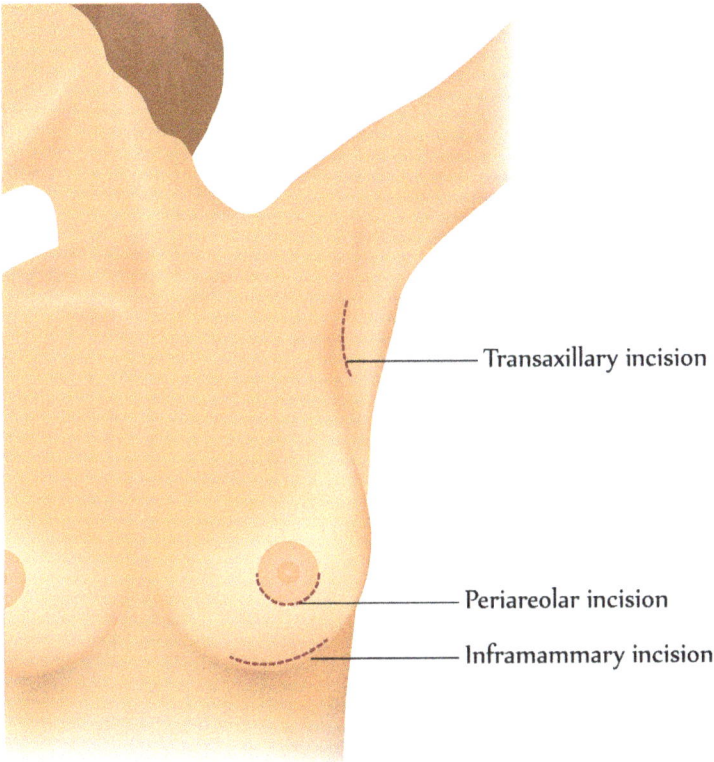

Transaxillary incision

Periareolar incision

Inframammary incision

There are some things to consider when you make your decision on the incision site for your augmentation:

If you wear a two-piece bathing suit, the IMF incision will be visible when you raise your arms and your bathing suit top rises slightly. This incision is also visible when your bathing suit top does not completely cover the inframammary fold area.

The most visibly prominent area of the breast is the nipple-areola complex. The periareolar incision is visible when topless. If you form a poor scar or a hypertrophic scar, the scar will be in a very noticeable position. Also, this approach is often associated with loss of sensation in the nipple area around the scar and a slightly higher risk of infection.

The transaxillary No Scar on the Breast incision is placed in the armpit, not the breast. In the unlikely event that a bad scar should form, it is in a well-hidden place. The underarm area has natural creases, so the incision can be well hidden in a crease. Rarely does anyone look under your arm. In addition, the infection rate is lowest using this incision.

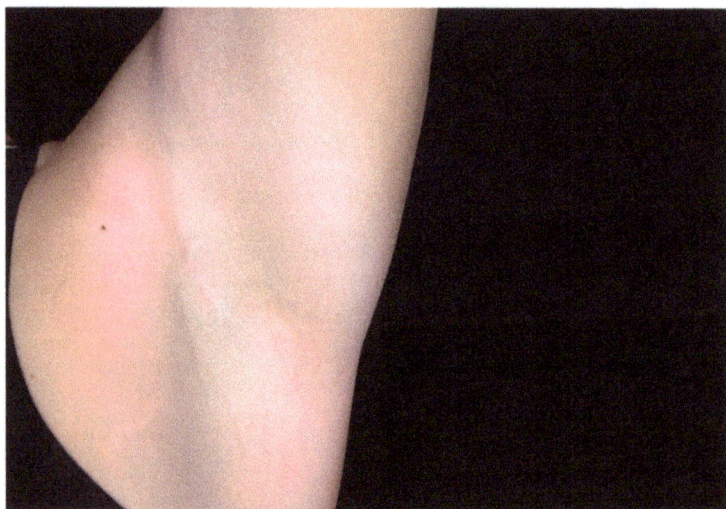

Note the well-healed incision that is "hidden" in the crease of the armpit and barely visible three months after surgery using the No Scar on the Breast technique.

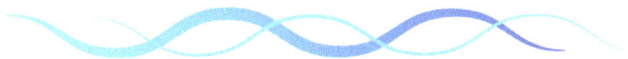

Q: **What are the advantages of the No Scar on the Breast transaxillary incision placement?**

A: With this technique there is no scar on the breast. Incisions placed in the inframammary folds beneath the breasts are visible in string bikinis or if the arms are raised when wearing a two-piece swimsuit. Incisions around the areola are visible when topless. The transaxillary technique leaves no evidence of surgery on the breast. The incisions are well hidden because the incision is placed in one of the natural creases in the underarm. If the scar is noticeable at all, most people don't associate a scar in the underarm with breast augmentation. Patients tell us they don't want a scar on the breast because they just don't want to have a reminder of a surgery, or any telltale signs that they've had some surgery. They want to get up in the morning, when they're getting dressed, look in the mirror and not see a scar.

This technique results in attractive, natural looking results. The armpit incision enables the surgeon to insert the breast implants beneath the chest muscle in an innovative "dual plane" placement. This placement provides a full, soft natural breast shape especially along the lower portion of the breast because the upper portion of the implant is hidden beneath the chest muscle and the lower portion lies directly beneath the breast tissue.

There is an option for either silicone or saline implants. Although some surgeons often limit patients to saline implants with the transaxillary approach, I routinely place silicone implants through the armpit as well. Another advantage of the underarm approach is that larger implants can be placed without worrying about the incision being stretched on the breast, or weakness in the breast gland such that the implant could push through.

Using this approach the patient has an easier recovery. When placing breast implants under the chest muscle, the transaxillary technique may make recovery easier than other techniques as the chest muscle can be "lifted" to insert the implant instead of being cut. Breast tissue is also not cut with this technique. Incisions that are not under tension normally heal more rapidly. Incisions around the areola or in the breast crease can be under pressure from the implant itself. The armpit incision location is not subject to tension from the weight and projection of the implant.

There is also a lower risk of infection with the transaxillary technique. Use of this approach avoids the breast glands and nipples where there's generally a higher amount of bacteria that can cause infection.

With the inframammary fold approach, especially in women with a slightly droopy breasts, there can be bacteria along the skin due to the moisture in the area. We use a Keller Funnel™ to place the implants without direct contact, further reducing the risk of infections.

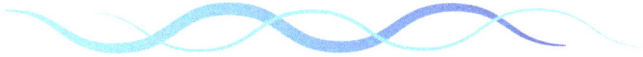

Q: *Patients that have excess skin or sagging of the breasts may be candidates for a breast lift, or mastopexy, along with augmentation. Mastopexy procedures require an incision in the inframammary fold at the bottom of the breasts. Would augmentation be performed using the inframammary fold incision in this case?*

A: A breast lift is performed to remove stretched skin and to renew the breast shape, without, by itself, increasing breast volume and projection. Both inframammary fold and periareolar incisions are typically used for a breast lift. It is possible that the inframammary incision will be used to insert the implants; however, many times we will still put in the implants through the underarm position for some technical reasons.

A breast lift (mastopexy) and augmentation can be performed at the same time. When performed through the mastopexy incisions on the lower breast, the breast tissues must be dissected in order to place the implant. In my opinion and the opinion of other surgeons with whom I have spoken, the dissection of the lower breast tissue weakens the supporting breast tissue and increases the chances of bottoming out of the breast implant. Bottoming out is a problem that is difficult to correct. Placing the implant through the underarm incision avoids dissection of the breast tissue and muscle from below. I have noted a lower incidence of bottoming out with this technique.

By going in through the underarm incision, we can place the implant beneath the muscle and under the breast gland in a dual plane position without weakening the breast tissue on the bottom of the breast.

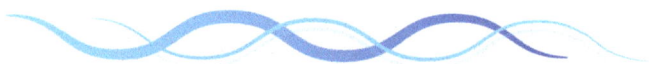

Q: The armpit is some distance from the breast. How are you able to accurately position the implants when inserting them from such a distance from the breasts?

A: Using technology that was originally developed for general surgery procedures inside the abdomen, we can accurately see into the area of the implant pocket and ensure that we get proper placement. We use an endoscope, which has flexible fiber optics to light the area and it has a camera attached that provides a 10X magnification image on a monitor. The magnified image allows us to clearly see the surgical field and to create a pocket that precisely fits the implant. With a magnified well-lit view of the pocket, we can ensure accurate placement of the implant. Additionally, we are able to look for any bleeding vessels. This results in a very low rate of bleeding after the surgery.

When using a periareolar incision or an inframammary fold incision, most surgeons only use a headlight or lighted retractor with no magnification. The technique using an endoscope is superior for viewing the implant pocket and detecting bleeding, so it can be stopped. Bleeding in the implant pocket is one of the major causes of capsular contracture. Detecting and thus being able to stop any bleeding is an important advantage of doing the transaxillary incision method using an endoscope.

We also use an innovative device to place the implant: the Keller Funnel™. This allows me to insert the implant into the pocket without directly touching the implant. The Keller Funnel™ not only makes it easier and safer to place implants through the shortest possible incision, but it also minimizes the risk of infection.

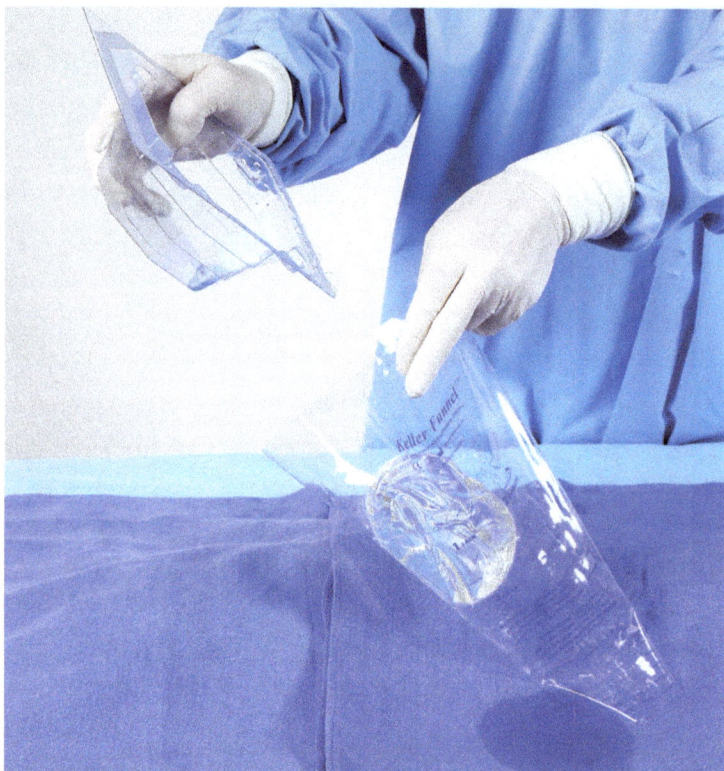

The Keller Funnel™ allows the surgeon to insert the implant without directly touching it, reducing the risk of infection.

Q: *What are the options for placement of the implants?*

A: We have two options for implant placement. The first method we call "dual plane submuscular," or "subpectoral" placement. With this placement the implant is inserted underneath the pectoralis muscle in the chest. Dual plane means the pectoralis muscle covers the top of the implant, and the implant lies beneath the fascia of the breast gland on the bottom half.

The second option is "subglandular" placement, where the implant is placed under the breast tissue, but on top of the pectoralis muscle in the chest. It is important to note that both of these placement options are available using the No Scar on the Breast technique. The image below shows the two placement options.

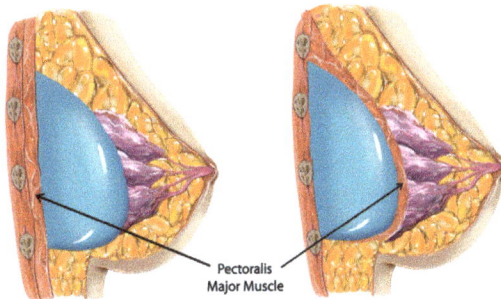

Pectoralis
Major Muscle

Subglandular Implant   Submuscular Impant
(Under the Breast Gland)   (Under the Pectoralis Major Muscle)

21

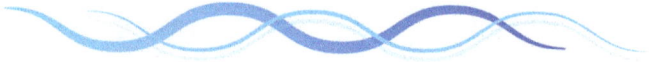

_Q:_ **_What are the advantages and disadvantages of_**
submuscular placement?

_A:_ With submuscular placement the results look more
natural because the chest muscle covers the implant.
For a patient who's very thin and doesn't have a
lot of breast tissue, going under the muscle is the
preferred approach because the muscle camouflages
the top edge of the implant. An analogy I use: if I
put a marble on a table and put a handkerchief over
it, you would say, "Hey, there's a marble under that
handkerchief." If I throw a thick blanket over it, you
would say, "Well, there's something there, but I can't
really tell what it is." When you have a thinner person
with very little breast tissue, especially in the upper
aspect of the breast, you don't have much tissue to
cover the implant. If you put an implant in over the
muscle, you're going to see the outline of the implant.
If the patient decides that's what she wants, we can
go over the muscle. If she says, "No, I really don't
want my implant to be noticeable," then we will have
to go under the muscle.

Risk of future breast sagging is diminished with
submuscular placement because the chest muscle
supports the implant. Mammograms are easier to

read with this approach and studies have shown that placing the implant beneath the muscle reduces the risk of capsular contracture.

Placement under the muscle allows the implant to move with flexing of the pectoralis muscles. Although this is not a motion women typically perform, body builders or women who use their chest a lot, like massage therapists, do flex their chest muscles. In such a case, they may find the motion of the implant not desirable, and may prefer to place the implant over the muscle.

Submuscular placement may result in a slightly longer recovery period and possibly more post-operative discomfort during recovery.

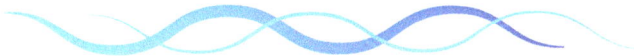

Q: **What are the advantages and disadvantages of subglandular placement?**

A: If a woman has enough breast tissue to cover the implant, then placement over the muscle and under the breast gland will generally have a good result. If the patient exercises her pectoralis muscles through exercise, such as with bodybuilding, or if her regular activities or work involves flexing the pectoralis muscles, this is a better placement option. As mentioned in the previous answer, implant placement under the muscle will result in movement of the implants with flexing of the pectoralis muscles. Many women find this motion to be undesirable. Subglandular placement also typically provides a shorter recovery time.

If a patient doesn't have enough breast tissue, this placement option may not yield natural looking results, as the implants may be more noticeable and an outline of the implant may be visible. Additionally, the breasts are more likely to droop in the future because the breast tissue is not as well supported. This also complicates any future breast lift procedures because the blood supply is removed from the pectoralis muscle to the overlying breast gland.

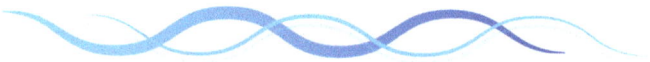

Q: What are the differences, advantages and disadvantages of silicone and saline implants?

A: Saline implants are filled with a sterile saltwater solution, similar to the fluid that is naturally present in the human body. They are placed into the implant pocket empty and are then filled through a valve. The surgeon can adjust the fill volume to achieve optimal results and they are a good choice for women with different sized breasts. Saline breast implants have been a popular option for a long time and they are available in a wide selection of sizes and shapes to accommodate different body types.

Saline implants give the breast a full, rounded look that adds greater volume to the breast. They give the breast a nice fullness at the top while maintaining the natural teardrop appearance. Since saline implants are filled with a saltwater solution, if a leak ever occurs, it will go "flat" and it will be very obvious to the patient. Saline implants will feel firmer than silicone implants. A limitation of saline implants is that the larger the implant and the less breast tissue a woman has, the more likely it will ripple or be felt underneath the skin, if using subglandular placement. As long as the patient has adequate breast tissue to cover the implant, saline implants can be an excellent choice. All saline implants are a round shape.

Silicone implants have become the implant of choice for most women since being re-introduced to general usage in 2006. Silicone implants are pre-filled with a silicone gel fluid that very closely resembles the feel of a natural breast. The new silicone gel implants are more cohesive and therefore less likely to leak into the tissues if ruptured. They offer a much softer feel compared to saline implants and they allow women with small breasts to have larger enhancements without the problems of rippling that can occur with saline implants. Silicone implants are offered in a wide variety of shapes and sizes including round and the anatomical teardrop shape.

There was a controversy with silicone implants back in the late '80s and early '90s, when the implants had a more 'liquid' form of silicon dioxide inside that could leak into the body tissue if the implant was ruptured. The real issue was the lack of purity of the silicon dioxide. The impurities in the silicone could leach out of the implant and in some cases caused women to feel bad. It took a while to understand the cause and once it was determined that the issue was with impurities, not the silicon dioxide itself, improved techniques were implemented in the manufacturing process to ensure the purity of the silicon dioxide. If fact, today every batch of silicon dioxide that will be used in implants must be tested for purity.

In 2006, after rigorous scientific review, the United States Food and Drug Administration (FDA) approved the marketing of the new silicone gel-filled implants for breast reconstruction in women of all ages and for breast augmentation in women ages 22 and older. I had been an investigator and was involved with the FDA-approved study allowing women to receive silicone breast implants since 1998.

Silicon dioxide is not toxic to humans. It's in our toothpaste; in our baking powder; it's in the environment. Silicon dioxide is used to make IV tubing, IV bags, pacemakers, joint implants, and other medical devices that are placed inside the body. All of the silicone implants currently being used are what we call cohesive. Even though the gel is soft, it is has a form, and if the implant shell were to crack, the silicone does not leak as it did with the older implants.

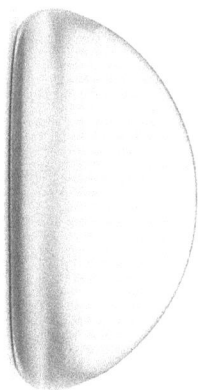

Round Silicone
Gel Implant

Teardrop "Gummy
Bear" Implant

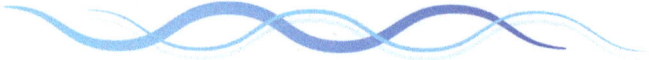

Q: **With so many options for shape and size of implant, how does a patient choose the right implant?**

A: It is important for the patient to convey to her surgeon what she is wanting for a result. Choosing an implant size can be one of the most difficult decisions for a woman planning for breast augmentation; however, there is typically a right size for each patient. The optimal size generally should be determined based on the width of the implant matching the width of the patient's breasts rather than the volume. As the implant gets larger in volume, the width becomes wider. It is important that the proper size and profile implant is chosen to ensure optimal result and optimal cleavage.

The most common shape for an implant is the round shape. If you hold up a round implant, it will take the shape of a teardrop and when you lay it flat, it flattens out like a breast. This shape provides the most natural appearance overall. Today, there are also anatomical shaped implants that are form-stable, meaning they don't change shape. Although some women choose this shape, and it looks good when you are standing or sitting, when you lay down, it retains its teardrop shape. A natural breast does not retain a teardrop shape when you lay down. That's why most patients prefer the round implants because they look more like a natural breast when you lay down or stand up.

I have found that showing patients a 3-D image of what they will look like with various implant options makes the decision much easier. State-of-the art 3-D imaging systems are very expensive and only a small fraction, about 10% of plastic surgeons, have made the investment in this revolutionary equipment. Our office has three 3-D imaging systems. I have found that being able to view the new you in 3-D before the surgery leads to greater patient satisfaction and their result is aligned with the image they were able to see in advance. We take a three dimensional image of the patient and then simulate what the augmentation is going to look like with different sizes and shaped implants. I put the image on a big screen to view. The image is in three dimensions. I can rotate the image into different angles to allow the patient to get an idea from different perspectives of what the result will look like.

We also have plenty of before and after pictures in our gallery that we can show patients. We can pick out past patients that look similar to them in the before pictures and then show the after pictures to get another idea of what they will look like after the procedure.

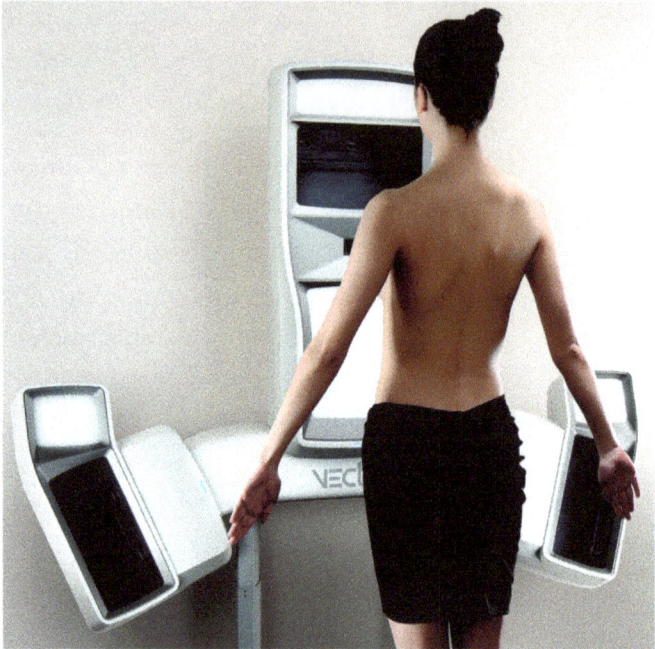

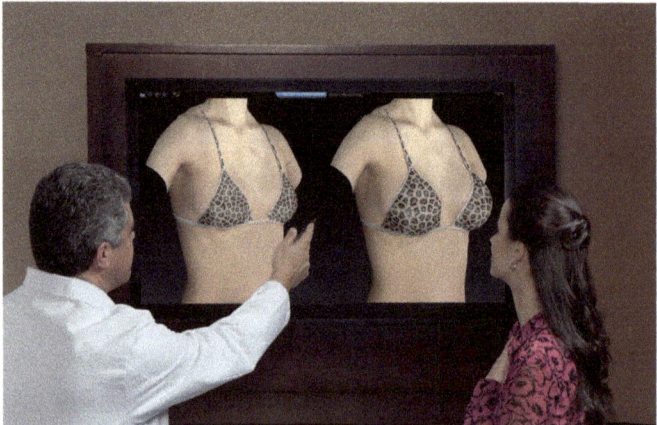

3-D imaging allows the patient to visualize what they will look like after their breast augmentation.

Q: *How long are today's implants expected to last? Do they come with a warranty?*

A: Quality levels and failure rates have improved dramatically since the 1980s. Current implant technology has improved to the point that they have a less than 10% failure rate after 10 years. Some studies will show as low as three, some as high as nine percent. There's always a very small chance that your implants could fail, and of course there's a great warranty. The implant manufacturers will replace your implant in the unlikely event of failure. However, the odds are now that if you have augmentation, 10 or 15 years later you're going to change out your implants not because of failure, but because your breast shape changes. The most frequent reason I have for implant exchange now is not because of failure, but because of a change in the shape of the breast as the woman ages and goes through breast altering changes. If you tend to lean down or you have babies, your breast volume is going to change, and you'll want to have your implants switched accordingly. You might need to go larger; you might go smaller.

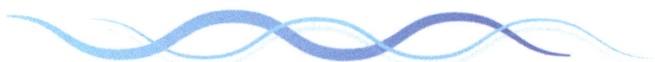

Q: *If a woman is interested in a breast augmentation procedure and doesn't want to be left with a scar on the breast, how should she select a qualified plastic surgeon?*

A: To successfully perform a breast augmentation procedure using the transaxillary approach, where the incision is made in the armpit, the plastic surgeon must be experienced in endoscopic surgery. Less than 20% of plastic surgeons in the United States have the training and have invested in the equipment necessary for this type of surgery. Even fewer have substantial experience in proficiently performing this technique. Patients are advised to look for a plastic surgeon that has a reputation for doing augmentation on a regular basis, and then has demonstrated experience with the transaxillary incision approach to breast surgery where scarring of the breast is avoided. Research can be done by asking friends for recommendations, talking to people who have actually had the surgery, by searching the Internet for surgeons specifically experienced in this approach, and also by reviewing online ratings.

During consultation, some plastic surgeons may say that the patient is not a good candidate for a transaxillary approach, even though the patient clearly is a good candidate. The reason may be that the surgeon doesn't know how to do it. If you want your breast augmentation without a scar on the breast, make sure you are consulting with a surgeon that has significant experience with this approach; otherwise you may not receive appropriate advice.

I mentioned earlier about the benefits to the patient if they can see a simulation of their results in advance with 3-D imaging, so it is also recommended to seek a plastic surgeon that has the advanced 3-D imaging system. The patient's ability to imagine what their results will look like with various implant types, sizes and shapes significantly reduces uncertainty about the expected result.

Having good communications and rapport with the surgeon is also important for an overall good experience for the patient. Patients can get a great result through any incision, but working with a surgeon that has a similar thought process can provide a thorough understanding of the procedure, answer your questions, and explain what you will be getting into. This will make for a much happier experience. You should be able to have a good feeling that you are compatible with your surgeon during your consultation.

Finally, make sure that your surgeon is Board Certified by the American Board of Plastic Surgeons.

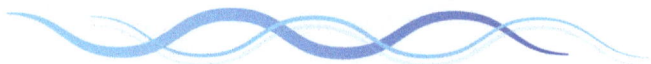

Q: Since the transaxillary incision approach most often provides a higher level of patient satisfaction since no scar is left on the breast, why aren't more plastic surgeons using this technique?

A: When a new medical technique becomes available, it takes a number of years before it becomes widely utilized. It was only in the early to mid-1990s that plastic surgeons were starting to consider using fiber optic assisted breast augmentation through an underarm incision. Before that time there were no professors who knew how to use this technique and so younger plastic surgeons were not being trained in the procedure.

Even though endoscopic surgery has been around for some time now, it's a more technologically advanced procedure. The surgeon has to be comfortable using the fiber optic devices; be able to use their hands in one direction while looking at a monitor in another. It's like working with robotics and some surgeons can't do it; they have to look directly at what they're working on.

The other reason is the market and the competition. If the surgeon is getting good results doing inframammary fold or periareolar incisions and no one else in the market is doing transaxillary incisions, they most likely are not going to go back to learn another way to do it.

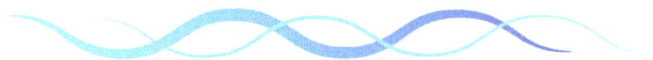

Q: **What is recovery like after a No Scar on the Breast augmentation procedure?**

A: In the first three or four days, you're going to have limitations on range of motion of your arms, because when you raise your arm or move it outward, you're going to stretch the pectoralis muscle. That will go away over a period of three to four days and most patients are then able to perform typical activities of daily living. Initially, the breasts will be swollen and they'll have a slightly distorted shape. They'll be bruised and swollen for the first week to two weeks. In the second and third week, you'll start to see the shape of the breast improving. Around three weeks, most people are pleased with the shape of their breast and feel comfortable in an outfit that shows cleavage. At about six to eight weeks, people are very pleased because that's the time when the skin has relaxed and the breast starts to look more like a natural breast.

Patients who have a desk job, or a job that doesn't require a lot of chest activity, could go back to work in five to seven days. For someone who does a lot of physical activity, pushing and pulling type motions, they may need about 10 to 12 days. Someone who's a fitness instructor or lifts a lot of heavy weight are not going to be able to do chest motions for about six to eight weeks. Other motions they could do. Physically active women can run as soon as they feel comfortable running. High impact activities cause a little bit of jarring of the breast, and so it's sore in the first week to two weeks. Most women feel comfortable running from two weeks on. Prior to the two weeks, if they want to get some kind of cardiovascular workout, they can do some low impact activity such as riding a stationary bike to avoid the impact and the bouncing motion that would cause the breast to be sore.

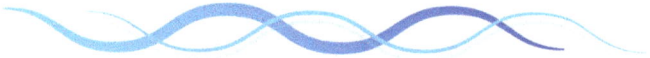

Q: ***What are the risks of breast augmentation surgery?***

A: As with any surgery, there is always the risk of infection, but that's very low. We perform surgery in an operating room with a very sterile environment and I have yet to have a primary breast augmentation infection. Capsular contraction, or formation of scar tissue around the implant, when thickened, can make the implant feel hard and round. Surgeons who do this on a regular basis will have a low capsular contracture rate and our experience is less than 1%. The submuscular position of the implants provides the least risk for capsular constriction. Risk of post-operative bleeding is also very low and is more likely to occur if the patient has an accident soon after surgery.

Before And After Pictures

Below are **_actual_** before and after photos of two of Dr. Burden's breast augmentation patients.

In both cases, silicone gel implants were placed using the "No Scar on the Breast" technique. Note that there is no scar in the fold that can be seen topless. There is also no scar around the areola that is a telltale sign of surgery.

Readers can see an extensive gallery of Dr. Burden's patients' before and after breast augmentation photos by visiting:

www.ThePlasticDoc.com

Patient 1

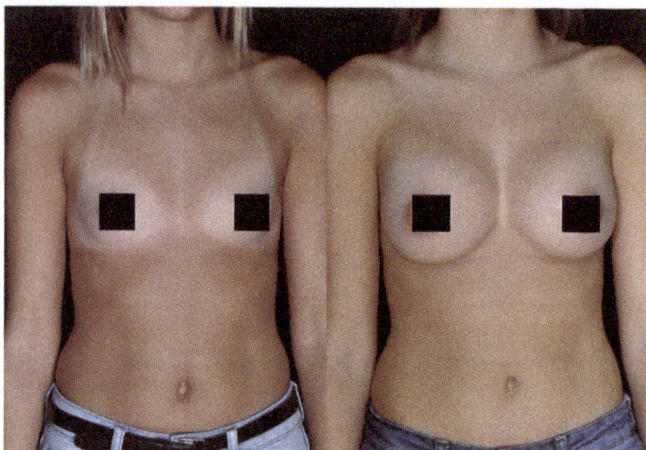

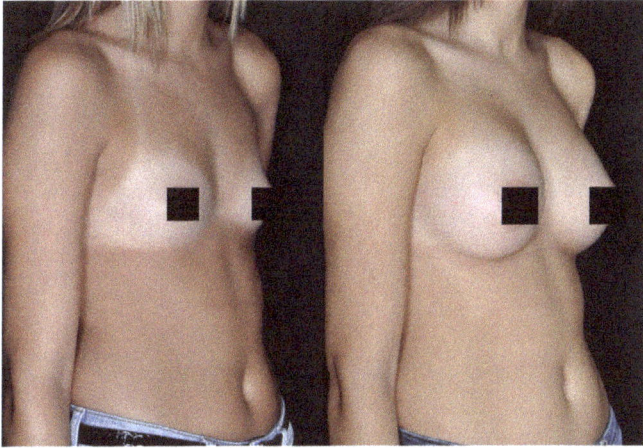

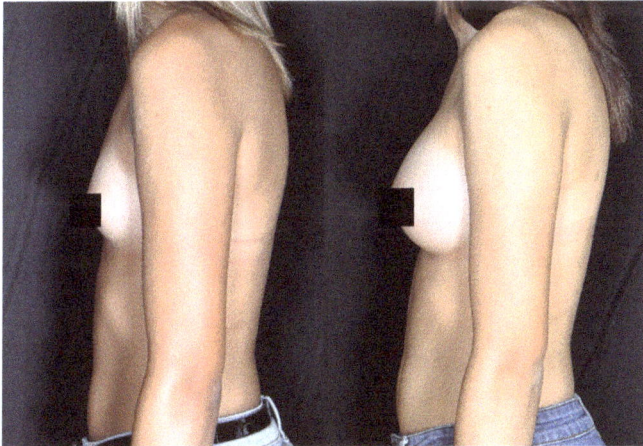

Patient 2

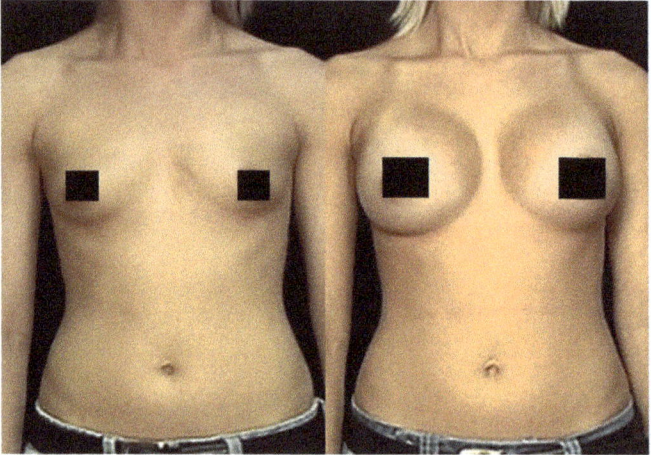

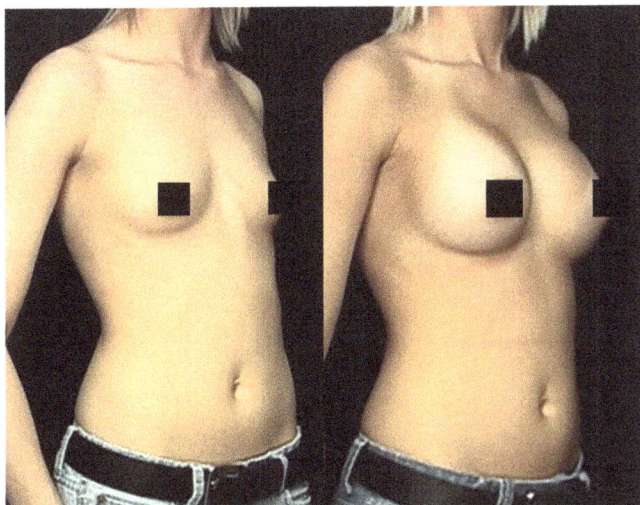

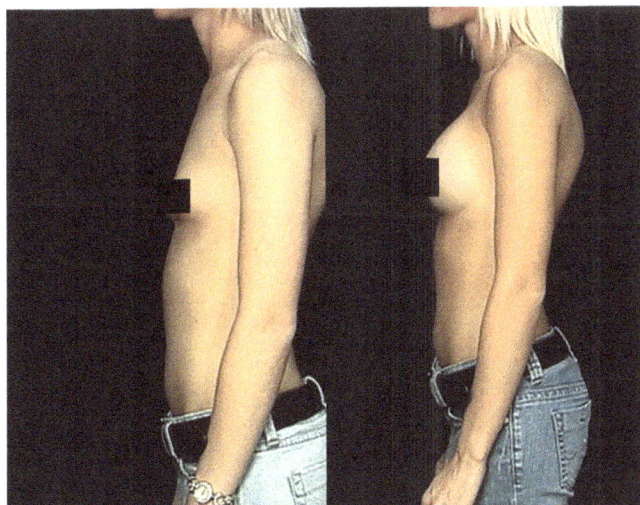

What Patients Are Saying

"*Dr. Burden,*

Thank you so much!!! I love my new look after my breast augmentation surgery this past summer. I am amazed at how natural they look and feel. I had a wonderful experience, surgery went great and it was nothing. I was expecting the worst and it was a piece of cake! All your staff were so kind, helpful and professional. Thank you, thank you!!! I am so happy, it's a NEW ME!"

- K.E., Memphis, TN

"*Dr. Burden and Staff,*

I wanted to tell you all thank you for the wonderful care I received. You truly changed my life!"

S.M., Pensacola, FL

"Thank you Dr. Burden for excellent communication skills. I was so impressed with the amount of time you spent with me during the consultation. All of my questions were answered without making me feel rushed through the office. I see now why Destin Plastic Surgery has an excellent reputation."

- B.P., New Orleans, LA

"Dear Dr. Burden,

In November of 2007, you performed this procedure (breast augmentation) on me. They are beautiful. I recently had my gyn. check up with my doctor and I had to tell him of my surgery. He could not believe there were NO incision marks anywhere. Even after I showed him where they were he was amazed because they had healed up so well that you cannot tell I ever had surgery! I took that as a great compliment because he has been in practice for many, many years and he has seen many breast procedures. It actually appears that mine are perfectly grown that way! WOW! Thank you so much. I was 45 years old and married for 25 years before I had it done and it has been such a catalyst for me wanting to take really good care of myself. I walk several miles a day and pay attention to the kinds of food I put into my body. I actually make ME a priority which I always had a hard time doing. Many thanks again to you and your wonderful staff!"

- Sincerely, L.B., Ozark, AL

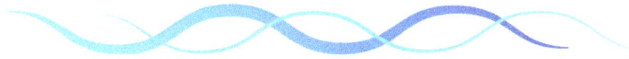

"Dr. Burden,

I wanted to take the time to thank you and your staff for an excellent experience. From my initial consultation to follow-up visits, I have always felt that I was in the very best of hands. Everyone has been extremely professional, caring and attentive to all of my needs and concerns. Thank you so much for huge positive change you've made in my life."

-K.C., Pensacola, FL

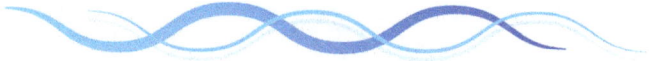

"Hello Dr. Burden,

My wife recently had breast augmentation at your facility about a week or so ago, and I just wanted to thank you for such a wonderful job that you did for my wife. Her expectations were exceeded by your expert work and knowledge. Your entire staff there is absolutely first class, and each and every member there was very kind and administered the kindest and most utmost care that you don't usually receive at the medical facilities here in Atlanta.

Once again thank you, and we hope to be back soon to see you for some more consultations in the future."

- C.C., Atlanta, GA

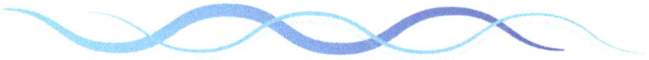

"Dr. Burden, Joan, & Staff,

I wanted to say that my experience with each of you from start to finish was nothing short of outstanding. You are truly a First Class, World Class operation and you treat your patients the same. Every *question--no matter how small--was addressed quickly and kindly. And, every step of the process was so well laid out and processed seamlessly through the operation on to after-care. I could not praise you both enough for your amazing gifts and abilities you shared with me along with the others who assisted from start to finish. Proud to say I had the pleasure first hand of changing my life in your amazing care. Thank you!"*

-D.S., Jackson, TN

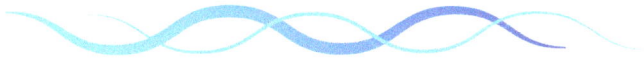

"Dr. Burden- *I would just like to let Dr. Burden know that he and his staff are excellent and I appreciate everything you have done for me... and Joan is the best person that we as patients can ask for...she is an excellent nurse as well as a perfect person...thx a lot for great care."*

- T.C., Pace, FL

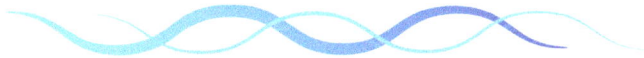

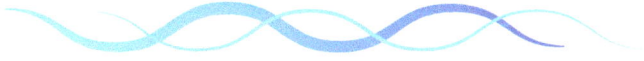

About The Author

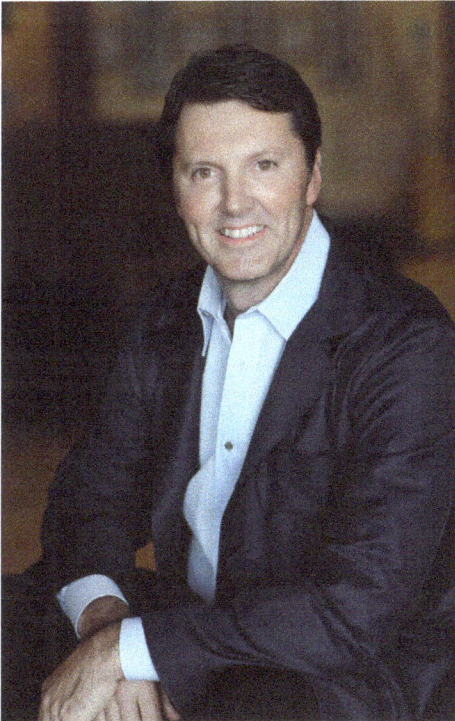

William R. Burden, M.D., F.A.C.S., is a Board Certified Plastic Surgeon, a Fellow of the American College of Surgeons and a member of the American Society of Plastic Surgeons. He is the founder and CEO of Destin Plastic

Surgery in Destin, Florida, one of the Southeast's most recognized cosmetic facilities. He is also the founder of the Destin Surgery Center, housed in the same building.

While in high school, Dr. Burden took anatomy classes offered at the Medical College of Virginia on the weekends. He also took classes in Medical Genetics and Computer programming. Because of high PSAT and SAT scores, he was selected to attend college classes prior to graduating from high school at Virginia Tech.

Dr. Burden received his Bachelor of Science in Biochemistry from Virginia Tech and his Medical Degree from the Medical College of Virginia. While at Virginia Tech, he was involved in genetics research. At the Medical College of Virginia, he was involved in Vitamin A research and its role in cancer prevention.

Dr. Burden completed his residency in General Surgery at Louisiana State University School of Medicine. While there, he authored several papers and was involved in vascular surgery research and spinal cord injury research.

While in his fellowship in Plastic Surgery at the University of Florida, Dr. Burden worked with his professors to introduce endoscopic techniques in breast surgery and specialized microvascular techniques for breast and body reconstruction.

During his fellowship at the University of Florida, Dr. Burden was one of the pioneers in researching the use of endoscopic or fiber optic technology for plastic surgery. He saw the potential for use of this new technology to enable accurate placement of breast implants using an incision in the underarm area instead of on the breast.

Dr. Burden's vision was to perfect a procedure using the latest technology that would provide the best results in terms of breast augmentation without leaving a visible scar on the breast. Although some breast augmentations had been done by plastic surgeons using an incision in the armpit prior to this time, the ability to accurately dissect and place the implants was a limiting factor in the use of this technique. During the course of his fellowship, Dr. Burden and the team he was working with were successful in achieving his vision.

When Dr. Burden entered private practice, he offered the transaxillary approach, with the incision in the armpit along with the more traditional approaches to breast augmentation. Even though all of the approaches to breast augmentation can provide good results in terms of breast volume and shape, over time, he found that the highest patient satisfaction level was achieved when the patient had no scar on the breast.

Dr. Burden is known nationally and internationally for the No Scar on the Breast procedure. He has been performing the No Scar on the Breast procedure for over twenty years and has completed thousands of No Scar on the Breast surgeries.

Women travel from across the country and from around the world to have their procedures performed by Dr. Burden. Among his patients are Miss USA and Miss America contestants, country music performers and bathing suit models, to mention a few. In addition to breast augmentation, Dr. Burden performs a full range of cosmetic and reconstructive surgical procedures on the face and body. He has appeared on news reports for his expertise with the Brazilian Buttlift, facelifts, and eyelid surgery.

Dr. Burden has been on the Mentor Corporation advisory panel for both breast augmentation and breast reconstruction. He is also on the Allergan Corporation advisory panel for new technology in breast augmentation and for their facial aesthetics and injectables products. He is a member of the Allergan Speaker Bureau and instructs and educates other physicians, nurses, and medical personnel on facial aesthetic treatments. In addition, he has participated in the national study for the reintroduction of the silicone gel implant.

Dr. Burden's surgeries are conducted at the Destin Surgery Center, co-located with Destin Plastic Surgery. The center is fully accredited by the Accreditation Association for Ambulatory Health Care and was ranked as one of the best hospitals by *US News and World Report*. Over 16,000 procedures have been performed at this facility. A full-time attending anesthesiologist is the Medical Director of Destin Surgery Center.

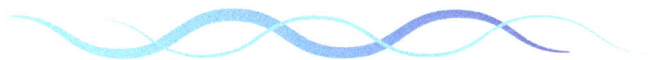

For More Information

For more information about Dr. William Burden and breast augmentation with the No Scar on the Breast procedure, visit:

http://www.ThePlasticDoc.com

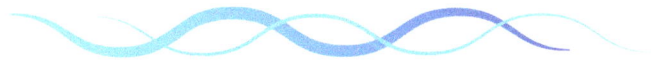

CONTACT INFORMATION

Destin Plastic Surgery

The Grant Building
4485 Furling Lane
Destin, Florida 32541

Phone: (850) 654-1194

Toll-free: (866) ENHANCE (364-2623)

Glossary

Breast Augmentation: In general, this surgical procedure is performed to increase breast volume and improve breast shape with implants.

Capsular Contraction: Capsular contraction, or formation of scar tissue around the implant, when thickened, can make the implant feel hard and round. Submuscular positioning of the implants provides the least risk for capsular constriction.

Dual plane submuscular implant placement: A "dual plane submuscular," or "subpectoral" implant is one of two implant placement options. With this placement, the implant is inserted underneath the pectoralis muscle in the chest. "Dual plane" means the pectoralis muscle covers the top of the implant, and the implant is beneath the fascia of the breast gland on the bottom half.

F.A.C.S.: F.A.C.S. is an abbreviation which stands for Fellow of the American College of Surgeons.

FDA: FDA is an abbreviation which stands for the United States Food and Drug Administration (FDA).

Inframammary Fold (IMF) implant placement: In the inframammary fold (IMF) procedure, the implant is placed in the crease beneath the breast.

Keller Funnel™: An innovative device used to insert the implant into the pocket without directly touching the implant. The Keller Funnel™ not only makes it easier and safer to place implants through the shortest possible incision, but it also minimizes the risk of infection.

No Scar on the Breast procedure: The transaxillary No Scar on the Breast incision is placed in the armpit, not the breast. In the unlikely event that a bad scar should form, it is in a well-hidden place. The underarm area has natural creases, so the incision can be well hidden in a crease. Rarely does anyone look under your arm. In addition, the infection rate is lowest using this incision.

Periareolar incision: A periareolar incision runs along the lower border of the areola.

Saline implants: Saline implants are filled with a sterile saltwater solution, similar to the fluid that is naturally present in the human body. They are placed into the implant pocket empty and are then filled through a valve. The surgeon can adjust the fill volume to achieve optimal results.

Silicone implants: Silicone implants are pre-filled with a silicone gel fluid that very closely resembles the feel of a natural breast. The new silicone gel implants are more cohesive and therefore is less likely to leak into the tissues if ruptured. They offer a much softer feel compared to saline implants and they allow women with small breasts to have larger enhancements without the problems of rippling that can occur with saline implants. Silicone implants are offered in a wide variety of shapes and sizes including round and the anatomical teardrop shape.

Subglandular implant placement: "Subglandular" placement, where the implant is placed under the breast tissue and on top of the Pectoralis muscle in the chest.

Subpectoral implant placement: A "dual plane submuscular," or "subpectoral" implant is one of two implant placement options. With this placement, the implant is inserted underneath the pectoralis muscle in the chest. "Dual plane" means the pectoralis muscle covers the top of the implant, and the implant is beneath the fascia of the breast gland on the bottom half.

Transaxillary incision approach: With this technique there is no scar on the breast. Incisions placed in the in inframammary folds beneath the breasts are visible in string bikinis or if the arms are raised when wearing a two-piece swimsuit. Incisions around the areola are visible when topless. The transaxillary technique leaves no evidence of surgery on the breast. The incisions are well hidden because the incision is placed in one of the natural creases in the underarm. If the scar is noticeable at all, most people don't associate a scar in the underarm with breast augmentation.

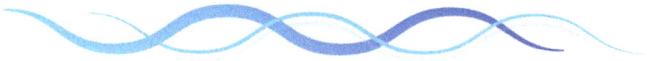

Notes